The All-Natural Cure for Your PMS

Summer 2007 Edition

By Andrew P. Jones, M.D.

ISBN 978-1-59916-272-0

Table of Contents

Introduction... 3

How Common Is PMS?................................. 9

Do YOU Have PMS? 15

What is PMS?.. 18

Modern PMS Theories 21

What Is the REAL Cause of PMS?................ 27

Sex Hormones – The Silent Culprit.............. 34

The Natural Hormones Dilemma –
Why Doctors Get Confused........................... 38

The Wild Yam Goose Chase.......................... 43

THE CURE: How to SUCCESSFULLY
Treat PMS.. 45

Neptune Krill Oil – Nature's Remedy
from the Sea 57

The Secret Mineral that Will Boost the
Effectiveness of Your Program and What
No Pharmacist Will Tell You about It............. 61

THE PLAN: Exact Dosages and Administration.................................... 65

THE SOURCES: Finding The Products – Quickly and Easily............................... 81

Summary of Recommendations – At a Glance 98

What to Do if All Else Fails? – (The "20%") 99

Conclusion... 116

Introduction

Congratulations – On the purchase of my book that will help you to end your PMS forever. You have taken the first step towards living a PMS-free life.

PMS is controversial. Many people and doctors have definite opinions on them, but exceedingly few offer up anything for curing it. They can't cure it because they don't know how to. But I do – and I have been curing PMS for a long time. Read on and learn exactly how you can cure your PMS once and for all.

If you are like my typical patient, you have been to 20 or 30 doctors over the years and taken numerous prescription medications. You have been prescribed anti-depressant medications, mainstream medicine's favorite remedy.

By now, you recognize these brand name anti-depressants: Effexor, Zoloft, Lexapro, Celexa, Paxil, Elavil, Zyban, Desyrel and the list goes on. They all have one thing in common: they don't work. Plus they just made you sleepy, lethargic and turned you into a drug dependent zombie.

The treatment is worse than the condition. In this case, the anti-depressants that doctors are so fond of prescribing forced you to make a choice between going off what your doctor recommended and returning to the PMS condition that was at least, drug free, or living like a zombie (and still suffering from PMS symptoms).

There is another group of women who have been searching the internet and libraries for years trying to find a solution to their PMS. Most likely you have come across information, much of it learned over a 50 year period.

This information touted bio-identical progesterone as the sole cure for PMS. Actually, they were very close and in many cases, natural progesterone (or bio-identical progesterone – same thing) worked like a charm. You used over the counter progesterone creams and literally took a bath in the creams, but they helped.

The problem was that even though the progesterone creams helped, you still had some residual effects from PMS. It just didn't quite go away completely liked you hoped.

Well, I have a cure. And it is very simple and straightforward. It relies on learned experience from the progesterone creams and from combining other known factors observed from patients with PMS. The combination of multiple variables results in a stunning success rate for eliminating PMS.

The treatment I recommend is safe. It is completely natural and will be described in detail later in this e-book. It is also inexpensive and has no unpredictable and unpleasant side effects. And nobody, I mean nobody, is out there in the mainstream medical community pursuing this avenue of treatment and cure.

What makes my approach to the cure of PMS even better is the fact that most people have many symptoms above and beyond PMS that affect them. For example, many women have painful menstrual cycles, or migraine headaches, or even infertility issues that most doctors do not even ask about when a woman comes in to see them complaining about her severe PMS.

All of these total body symptoms are related to one another in a big picture scenario that virtually all specialists in today's American medicine setting will miss. The narrow specializing doctors that people suffering with PMS are usually referred to have no idea about the relationship between these seemingly unrelated symptoms that are, in fact, all part of the same SINGLE problem.

The good news is that in my 18 years of private practice, I have managed to spend a lot of time with my patients and have asked a lot of questions about various health problems that were seemingly unrelated to the issues they have originally come to see me for. Having accumulated those years worth of observations, I have been able to put all of them together and discover that all of these symptoms are actually just consequential results from the same single problem.

For example, when we talk about PMS, the classic description you have probably heard has to do with a deficiency of natural progesterone. I will go on and discuss this in much more detail later in this book, but let's say this mechanism is completely accurate. (It is!). What then?

The secret is how to deliver to the body the most effective means to replenish the deficiency of natural progesterone and other metabolites that your body needs.

The answers are to follow.

An interesting story from the history books of medicine is the disease called scurvy. Three hundred years ago, crewmembers on ocean going ships sailed for months at a time on the open sea living off dry foodstuffs and fish. They had no fruit or vegetables. Many sailors were afflicted by scurvy, which is basically a severe deficiency of vitamin C.

Eventually, the British Navy figured out that if the crew were to eat limes during their long journeys that they would not get scurvy. It took three centuries to figure out the science, but they empirically noted it and treated the problem. Nowadays, every school kid in the world knows that vitamin C is found abundantly in fruit and even a small amount prevents scurvy.

The same type of approach follows for PMS. People do not get PMS because they are deficient in Effexor® or Imitrex® drugs. They get it because their bodies are deficient in certain substances called hormones. Later on I will tell you which ones in particular.

Read on for the most unique approach you have ever seen towards PMS. Actually, this approach I employ was standard medical treatment more than 60 years ago. This was before the days when lab tests took over all diagnostics and moved the physician from asking questions, to just ordering tests and letting the tests tell him what was wrong.

The problem with the modern medicine approach is that most of the time, lab tests are not helpful enough. The ranges for "normal" are so wide and the fact that the body can compensate so well on the last 10 percent of a functioning organ mean that lab tests are virtually always normal except in people who are ready for the hospital or the early grave.

By then, the lab tests are usually too late. Modern medicine needs to return to its roots just like the British Navy doctors did – by observation. Although we may not have the exact scientific mechanism to explain to the smallest detail what causes PMS, we can certainly employ the powers of observation and use what works to eliminate them altogether – for good.

Now, YOU will be the beneficiary of this approach. Just like the British Navy made its observations over the years and found out just how to prevent scurvy in its sailors, my progressive medical colleagues and I have discovered the **NATURAL SOLUTION** for curing PMS preventing it from happening in the first place.

How Common is PMS?

Depending on whose statistics you use, PMS is found in 75 – 80% of women. Women tend to experience PMS more frequently as they get older. Teenage girls tend to not complain about it as much, but that changes dramatically as a woman enters her late 20's and early 30's.

In fact, so many women have PMS that a woman who never experiences it is almost considered abnormal! Please remember that as recently as 20 years ago, mainstream medicine refused to even acknowledge the existence of PMS.

In the earlier days of the twentieth century, women were labeled as "hysterical" who complained of menstrual mood changes. This is what literally gave birth to the enormous size of the anti-depressant medication industry. This is why anti-depressants continue to be the most widely prescribed medications on the planet.

Only in the last two decades has mainstream medicine acknowledged that PMS exists and that it is indeed a true "physical" condition. It took 30 years of brushing women off as hypochondriacs before the paternalistic approach gave way to recognition that PMS is indeed a significant condition that affects tens (possibly hundreds) of millions of women, not just in the U.S., but worldwide.

Earlier studies raised the issue that Asians experience far less PMS than Westerners. However, recent surveys seem to refute this finding. This is interesting – because it would seem to indicate that PMS is a universal human (female) condition and not cultural or developmental phenomena.

PMS is Much More Common Than Realized

In real practice however, my observations have shown that PMS is even more common in the general population than formerly reported. This means that the 80% figure actually underestimates the true nature. In my observation, PMS is nearly universal approaching 100% of the female population whereby a woman will experience PMS will experience PMS at least one time in her life.

My actual experience is that far more women experience PMS tied to menstrual cycle changes than officially recognized. In all likelihood, this is due to external stimuli affecting the body – such as birth control pills, environmental toxins and certain prescription medications.

PMS Swelling Worldwide

What's even worse, PMS seems to be increasing worldwide, especially over the last 50 years, and particularly in women. Preliminary observations indicate that virtually every family in America has at least one female member experiencing PMS.

Mainstream medicine has speculated the reasons for the increasing incidence of PMS as four-fold:

- "Stress "
- A rise in the number of single-parent households
- An increase in the number of women in the workforce
- An increase in women who are dieting for weight loss

The Women's Health Institute of Texas believes in alternate explanations for the increasing incidence of PMS:

- Increased use of birth control pills since 1960
- Progressive exposure to "xenoestrogens" over the last 50 years
- Worsening dietary habits over the last 25 years

All three reasons certainly account for the disturbing uptrend in PMS. The entire population is being exposed to high levels of xenoestrogens, and the dietary habits of both men and women have progressively declined - as evidenced by the ever-rising numbers in obesity.

Part of the dietary changes include the nutritional devaluation of the food supply. A proliferation of antibiotics and hormones added to animal feed ends up on your dinner plate. Also decades of soil depletion of crop farm land has led to a bankruptcy of nutrients and minerals in grains, fruits and vegetables.

What are Xenoestrogens?

Xenoestrogens are chemicals exhibiting estrogen-like activity. Estrogen is one of the main female hormones. "Xeno" means foreign, so xenoestrogen simply means "a foreign estrogen." There are tens of thousands of chemicals that exert hormonal effects, with xenoestrogens exerting estrogenic effects.

Examples of xenoestrogens include pesticide residues on fruits and vegetables, hormone additives to grain fed beef and "gas off" from plastic water bottles.

Too much exposure to estrogen can cause numerous medical difficulties, manifesting as a myriad of "female" problems in women. These range from PMS, to uterine fibroids, to breast cancer. In men, these can range from gynecomastia (development of breast tissue) to prostate cancer.

Incidentally, this problem doesn't just involve humans. A recent article in "The Week" magazine cites estrogen-like contaminants being responsible for male fish in Maryland's Potomac River actually carrying eggs! What used to be a one in a million abnormality now affects 80% of the smallmouth bass population.

PMS used to be an uncommon condition a century ago. Today, PMS has become a worldwide epidemic representing a public health issue that authorities are missing out on.

PMS usually goes hand in hand with other "female" problems like migraine headaches, uterine fibroids, ovarian cysts, irregular and painful periods, post-partum depression and various cancers. Surgical procedures, like hysterectomies, are so commonplace that about a half million women are getting them done on an annual basis in the US alone. Worldwide, hysterectomies are probably numbering in the millions.

It is not natural that all of these problems are occurring. Migraines, PMS and hysterectomies are not normal and should not be considered so. Something is driving this trend – and it is getting worse, not better.

Birth control pills are a huge contributor to this epidemic, but public health exposure to xenoestrogens is sufficient enough by itself, to cause problems. The combination of effects from birth control pills and exposure to xenoestrogens is a catastrophe spiraling out of control.

But at least you are taking one small part of this into your hands. You can control some parts of this. The treatment program that you are about to learn will enable you to overcome and escape the pandemic that is occurring worldwide in women.

Read on and be free of PMS that has plagued you for so much in the past. Victory over PMS is imminent and in your grasp.

Do YOU Have PMS?

Here is how you can determine whether what you're experiencing is actually PMS:

> **If you experience any 3 or more of the following symptoms in the second half of your menstrual cycle, you are highly likely to have PMS:**
>
> - Mood swings
> - Crying spells
> - Depression
> - Insomnia
> - Anxiety
> - Weight gain
> - Breast swelling and tenderness
> - Abdominal distension and bloating
> - Water retention (edema – especially of ankles and feet)
> - Backache
> - Acne
> - Fatigue
> - Diarrhea
> - Constipation

> - Nausea
> - Parasthesias (electric tingling sensations)
> - Herpes – cold sores
> - Bruising easily
> - Joint pain (arthritis)
> - Muscle pain
> - Body aches
> - Poor concentration
> - Difficulty making decisions
> - Loneliness
> - Lethargy – increased need for sleep
> - Headaches – tension
> - Headaches – migraine
> - Cravings for salty foods

Typically these symptoms disappear rapidly with the onset of your period. Most women will not have all of these symptoms at the same time (heaven forbid!), but at some point or another in your life, most will experience nearly all of the symptoms.

This cycle gets repeated over and over every month for years or decades. As you well know, this becomes predictable and your whole family knows it. You know it even while you are experiencing it but there is nothing you can do about it.

Even the most disciplined of women with enormous self control are unable to control these symptoms.

This demonstrates the power of PMS and how hormones influence and control everything in your life.

If you are reading this e-book because of severe, debilitating PMS that are poisoning your life, do not respond to prescription medications, and keep coming back over and over again; you are in luck. And yes, it CAN be cured once and for all.

What is PMS?

Now that you have established that you really do have PMS, just what is PMS anyway? Ask 10 doctors and you will get 10 opinions. It just seems that nobody really knows.

PMS or "Pre-Menstrual Disorder" (now called Pre-Menstrual Dysphoric Disorder or PMDD in the medical community) is loosely defined as a cluster of symptoms that occur in the portion of your menstrual cycle just prior to the onset of menses. Hence the name, "re-Menstrual Disorder"

Now that the medical and scientific community has finally embraced PMS as an official "disease", they just couldn't stand to call it PMS. They had to give a fancy medical (psychiatric) name: PMDD.

If you really pin down the medical community on the naming of this condition, they tend to classify it as more of a psychiatric condition than a medical condition.

Mainstream medicine still just doesn't "get it".

Here are the symptoms commonly associated with PMS:

- Mood swings
- Crying spells

- Depression
- Insomnia
- Anxiety
- Weight gain
- Breast swelling and tenderness
- Abdominal distension and bloating
- Water retention (edema – especially of ankles and feet)
- Backache
- Acne
- Fatigue
- Diarrhea
- Constipation
- Nausea
- Parasthesias (electric tingling sensations)
- Herpes – cold sores
- Bruising easily
- Joint pain (arthritis)
- Muscle pain
- Body aches
- Poor concentration
- Difficulty making decisions
- Loneliness
- Lethargy – increased need for sleep
- Headaches – tension
- Headaches – migraine
- Cravings for salty foods

PMS is clearly related to your menstrual cycle. Timing is everything. These symptoms tend to cluster in the second half of your cycle which technically falls into the "post-ovulatory" phase.

Let's define the menstrual cycle. There is a lot of confusion over how you count days of your cycle. Day one is the first day of your period. Once you know how day one is counted you should never get confused.

Somewhere around day 14 is when you ovulate. This is right in the middle of your cycle. After this point is when the PMS symptoms begin. They start slowly, then gradually build up into a crescendo of symptoms in the days just prior to the onset of your period. Finally, they break off with relief with the arrival of your period.

Modern PMS Theories

There are a number of theories out there on what causes PMS. The most popular is the one formulated by Dr. Jonathon Lee about 40 years ago where he described a deficiency of progesterone occurring just prior to the onset of menses.

Another pioneer, Dr. Kathleen Dalton in England advocated the same theory and used herself as a guinea pig and self injected progesterone with good results. She also started injecting her patients with progesterone and also obtained good results for PMS type symptoms, as well as for resolving migraine headaches.

Very similar to the progesterone deficiency theory is the estrogen excess or estrogen dominant theory. Since hormones are present at the same time the presence of one hormone influences other hormones. An excess of one hormone may lead to a deficiency or simply an imbalance in the normal order of hormone strength.

So the estrogen excess theory states that excessive production or exposure to estrogen inhibits the actions of progesterone on the body. The estrogen dominance theory simply means that the balance of estrogen to progesterone is tipped in favor of estrogen thereby causing a disturbance of hormones in the body.

The net effect of the progesterone deficiency, estrogen excess or estrogen dominance theories are all the same: your progesterone is either not present in sufficient quantity, or is just being overpowered by estrogen.

I agree and concur with all of these theories. Mainstream medicine, however, does not. They love to cite studies showing that actually blood levels of estrogens and progesterone are "normal" in women with PMS.

They therefore conclude that since blood levels of hormones are normal, then hormones are not the cause of PMS. The same researches would likely conclude that the menstrual cycle is not hormonally related as well.

Intuitively, virtually every woman with PMS knows that this is a hormonally related disease, if for no other reason, that it is so consistent with the menstrual cycle.

The key to hormone levels is not to take mass readings from the population at large and then try to determine what range is "normal" or not. Rather the key is the hormonal variation within ONE woman. If your own hormone levels drop off, for whatever reason, then your own body senses a relative deficiency – and that is where the problems begin.

But when you show up at the doctor's office and have your hormone levels checked, they are always "normal". You are then dismissed as either hysterical or a hypochondriac, given a prescription for anti-depressant medications and dismissed.

I am certain this experience has happened to virtually every woman with PMS.

Other Theories

As far as other theories are concerned,, there are more influences on PMS than just the relative balance of estrogen and progesterone. Some have speculated that vitamin B6 is deficient as well as vitamin D deficiency.

Magnesium deficiency certainly contributes to hormonal symptoms, particularly since nearly a quarter of the population is deficient in magnesium. (More on magnesium deficiency later in this book).

There has been a very interesting study done in May of 2003 by the University of Montreal. They demonstrated that the administration of Neptune Krill Oil (NKO), which is a unique type of omega-3 fish oil had a significant improvement in PMS symptoms.

I have been an advocate of omega-3 oil (fish oil) for years. The demonstration of PMS improvement with Neptune Krill Oil should be considered a synergistic enhancement on the hormone responsiveness and not necessarily a cause, per se, of PMS.

There is a chemical in the brain called serotonin which impacts the mood symptoms of PMS. Serotonin is actually a hormone and mediates nerve cell transmissions. Researchers like to call serotonin a "neurotransmitter" for its role in mediating nerve to nerve communication in the brain and central nervous system.

Anti-depressant medications called "SSRI's" (Selective Serotonin Reuptake Inhibitors) affect the serotonin levels in the brain. These drugs work to inhibit the breakdown of serotonin, thereby increasing the amount of serotonin in the brain.

Anti-depressant medications like Celexa, Lexapro, Prozac, Paxil, Effexor and Zoloft are classical SSRI's. Virtually all of the modern anti-depressants fall into the SSRI classification. Older anti-depressants like Elavil and Wellbutrin are not SSRI's.

Doctors love to prescribe SSRI's for this very reason. Pharmaceutical companies also like it too. Perhaps the biggest reason Big Pharma is so profitable is because of the billions of dollars in SSRI prescriptions. Most of those prescriptions are for PMS and hormonally related problems, in my opinion.

Another hormone, called Prolactin, has been theorized as cause of PMS. Prolactin is the hormone that induces milk production after giving birth. This is the same hormone given to induce labor once your water has broken.

Finally, altered glucose metabolism has been offered for causing PMS. Altered glucose metabolism is extremely complex and may actually play a role. Unfortunately no one has figured out how to alter it in diabetes management very well.

Mainstream Medicine Theory

Currently, the mainstream medical community believes that serotonin and norepinephrine are the primary hormones involved in PMS. There is probably some truth to that theory and the medications they prescribe do indeed modulate the levels of those neurotransmitters.

But, my observations indicate that other hormones are involved as well.

Virtually every woman with PMS has some other type of a menstrual problem, like heavy and/or painful periods, irregular periods, migraine headaches, uterine fibroids, swelling, etc. Most have thyroid deficiency problems as well. The younger women may not manifest thyroid problems until after the birth of their first child. Infertility is another big problem on this list.

Many, if not most, women with PMS also tend to get worse after starting to take birth control pills. Women get temporary relief when they are pregnant.

All of this indicates that hormones, particularly the sex hormones in women, are strongly related to PMS.

What Is the REAL Cause of PMS?

OK, so I have teased you with the esoteric discussion of PMS causes and shown you all of the current theories. I have sprinkled in some of my observations. Now, you may rightfully ask, "Dr. Jones, can you just tell me what really causes my PMS?"

In the preceding chapter we have touched on the topic of hormones. We talked about the two favorite hormones of the medical establishment – serotonin and noreprinephrine. Mainstream medicine's favorite medications are those imposed upon them by the big drug companies – anti-depressants (Celexa, Lexapro, Prozac, Paxil, Effexor and Zoloft). They are selling huge dollar amounts of drugs to treat these serotonin and norepinephrine levels.

But – here is the **TRUTH**. The cause of PMS is NOT serotonin or norepinephrine (by themselves). It is not cortisone. It is not thyroid. There may be a significant relationship with estrogen, however. All of these are interrelated and play a role as they interact with one another, but they are NOT by themselves the root cause of PMS!

As stated earlier the overwhelming (90%) cause is a hormone called **PROGESTERONE**.

Actually, it is a deficiency of progesterone (or an imbalance in the ratio of progesterone and estrogen) that appears to be the root cause of PMS in women.

Stated another way, **it is an imbalance in the female sex hormones, progesterone and estrogen, that causes PMS**.

Earlier in 2006, the world's leading academic authority on migraine headaches (which are related to PMS) and their relationship to hormones, Dr. Vincent Martin of the University of Cincinnati College of Medicine, Ohio, published in the Journal, Headache, a blockbuster review article in which he discusses a theory called "estrogen withdrawal".

This is a variation of the progesterone deficiency theory. He noticed in a couple of studies done by earlier researchers that large quantities of estrogen administered late in the menstrual cycle that were suddenly withdrawn seemed to precipitate migraine headaches (and PMS).

This is precisely in the point of the menstrual cycle where progesterone is supposed to be produced in increasing amounts. When the progesterone fails to be produced in sufficient quantities, then the amount of estrogen that is still floating around is sensed by the body as excessive.

The levels of estrogen also fall off rapidly before the onset of menses. When this happens in an environment of insufficient progesterone, then this triggers PMS and migraine headaches.

Testing for Blood Levels of Hormones

When patients come into our clinic for an initial consultation and examination we have always tested for blood levels of multiple hormones: progesterone, testosterone, estrogen, cortisol and thyroid.

My medical colleagues and patients alike love to discuss various blood levels of hormones as if one were at an academy of science meeting with esoteric comments about a relatively higher or lower than normal result shown. But my observation has been that 95% of the time ALL blood testing is so-called "normal" – at least according to the laboratory's idea of what a normal range should be.

Hence the problem with blood level testing of hormones. They are nice to look at. They make a great source of conversation at follow-up doctor visits. But they really don't make a difference in the treatment plan.

In other words, they don't really affect the decisions or dosages in treating PMS. Regardless of how "normal" the blood testing is, we are still going to treat you the same way.

Why is this? Several reasons:

The lab's "normal" range is too wide. Virtually all labs consider one standard deviation "outside" the normal range. Mathematically, this puts 95% of the population in the "normal" range and only 5% of people as "abnormal".

If one considers the paradigm that 50% of women over the age of 35, for example, are deficient in progesterone, that stands to reason that the lab is missing an additional 45% or so of "abnormals".

What is more important - a lab's opinion of what your normal should be compared to a large population sample or what your own body considers to be a deficiency today relative to what your body experienced 10, 15 or 25 years ago?

In other words, the lab may say that you are "normal", whereas your body now has only half of the circulating progesterone (or estrogen, or thyroid) that you had when you were 20 years old.

What we don't have are the blood levels of what you had when you were 20 years old to compare back to. It is the relative difference inside your own body that makes all the difference.

So this is why blood testing is not important and not necessary in making recommendations for hormone replacement, at least in terms of managing PMS. And this is why as you read further on in my treatment recommendations that you will see nothing about getting blood tests or hormone levels checked.

The Other 10%

If progesterone deficiency is 90% of the cause of PMS, what about the other 10%?

This is where the interaction of hormones with other substances come into play. Hormones require a lot of interaction with other substances to make a desired physiologic reaction in the human body.

Magnesium Deficiency

For example, if there is a shortage of magnesium, then certain chemical reactions will either not occur or just be slowed down. Magnesium is required as a necessary co-factor in hundreds of chemical reactions within the body. A shortage of magnesium leads to problems.

Magnesium deficiency is extremely common in women with PMS and other hormonal problems. In the general population, you already stand a 40% chance of being deficient in magnesium.

Magnesium will be discussed later in this book in more detail, but we have observed that by the addition of magnesium with natural progesterone, we get an improved result for elimination of PMS symptoms.

Neptune Krill Oil (NKO)

The University of Montreal study on Neptune Krill Oil's (NKO) effects opened our eyes at the Women's Health Institute of Texas. We have previously been recommending fish oil as the official omega-3 supplement of choice, but when we changed over to NKO, the results improved when combined with natural sex hormones, thyroid and magnesium.

People, especially in Western society, do not get enough omega-3 oil in their diet. Omega-3 is found in concentrations 1000-fold higher in the brain than in the rest of the body. There are a number of studies linking omega-3 deficiencies and depression as well as a host of other problems.

For many years, omega-3 oils have been used by non-medical doctors to treat depression and other "mental health" conditions. There are some published studies on this with reported successes. However, we are not aware of any formal research using the combination therapy of omega-3 oils with the hormone replacements that we recommend.

Our clinical observations are that the combination of the hormones with the omega-3 greatly enhances the desired response of ending the depression. Therefore, our theory is that omega-3 oils have an interaction enhancing the effect of natural progesterone on the body.

Omega-3 oil has other uses as well. It is a wonderful natural anti-inflammatory agent. The bottom line is that we heartily endorse that everyone, male and female, take supplemental omega-3 supplements.

When we came across Neptune Krill Oil, we found that it is a better form of omega-3. It is absorbed by the body five or six fold better than standard omega-3 oils. NKO is one of the most powerful anti-oxidants on the planet. It is 47 times more potent as an anti-oxidant than standard fish oil.

As a result, we prefer NKO over standard fish oil preparations for the recommended omega-3 supplementation.

Now, let's take a closer look at **PROGESTERONE DEFICIENCY** in women.

Sex Hormones – The Silent Culprit

Progesterone is one of the main sex hormones in women. Actually, both men and women have progesterone circulating around in their bodies, but women just have a lot more of it.

Progesterone is a sex hormone produced largely by the ovaries. It is a counter-balance to estrogen, also largely produced by the ovaries. The adrenal glands can also manufacture sex hormones, but the ovaries are the primary production facility.

Progesterone and the other sex hormones are carried in the bloodstream all over the body. Every cell in the body, whether it is part of the uterus, heart, liver, eyeball or brain has a special progesterone receptor. This means that as progesterone (and all other hormones) are circulating throughout the body, every cell on every organ can be affected.

The sex hormones therefore are not just concerned with the sexual organs (uterus, breasts, ovaries, vagina), but all other organs are affected as well, especially the brain.

If there is a deficiency in progesterone, then every cell in every organ system can sense that. This is why a woman with a progesterone deficiency can have many, many different health issues. For example, a woman with a progesterone deficiency can have numerous problems with her menstrual cycle ranging from heavy periods to infertility. Virtually every woman with PMS has some menstrual problems as well.

The name Progesterone is derived from the base word – "gestation", or "pro gestation". This means that progesterone is responsible for the promotion and maintenance of pregnancy.

It is secreted by the ovary in the second half of the menstrual cycle. The menstrual cycle is typically 28 to 30 days long with the numbering system being the first day of menses counted as day one.

Days 1 through 7 are generally considered the period of menses where the levels of estrogen start to rise dramatically and progesterone level has already dropped off significantly. The lining of the uterus is sloughed off and the cycle begins anew.

Days 8 through 15 are concerned with selecting an egg (also called an ovum) and getting it ready for ovulation which occurs around day 14. During this time estrogen levels rise sharply and ovulation occurs with a spike of another hormone called Luteinizing Hormone or LH (which is the basis of the over-the-counter ovulation prediction kits sold in every pharmacy in the US).

Coincidentally, at the same time as ovulation a spike in the female levels of testosterone occurs. Testosterone is a known libido enhancer and I am certain that our species has been programmed to be especially receptive to sexual attraction around the time of ovulation.

The egg is ready for fertilization around day 14. The portion of the ovary responsible for that egg production is called the corpus luteum. This corpus luteum then begins to produce progesterone in large quantities in anticipation of a fertilized egg.

Days 15 - 22 or so result in a rapid and large increase in progesterone production. Once the body senses that the egg was not fertilized, then the progesterone component drops severely. The progesterone affects the lining of the uterus preparing it for a fertilized egg. The uterus gets enriched with blood vessels.

Once the progesterone level drops off, the overly enriched lining of the uterus sloughs off and the period begins anew, thus starting up the next cycle. A typical woman may have 400 cycles in her reproductive lifetime before this process gradually fades out into a menopausal state.

It is my observation that PMS symptoms are the most common during the time that the progesterone levels rapidly fall off. This is when mood swings, excessive swelling, breast tenderness, decreased libido, weight gain, and in some women, migraine headaches are at their peak.

My further observations of PMS in women include:

- ✓ the onset of PMS beginning with menarche (girls reaching puberty and beginning to have their first periods)

- ✓ onset or worsening of PMS with the administration of birth control pills.

- ✓ the relief of PMS during pregnancy

- ✓ the onset of PMS after the birth of the first child

- ✓ co-existence of PMS with migraines and depression

- ✓ correlation of PMS and post-partum depression – both due to crashing levels of progesterone

- ✓ the retention of PMS in post-menopausal women

- ✓ the worsening or prolongation of PMS in post-menopausal women with the administration of (HRT) Premarin ® and other chemically-altered estrogens.

Now, **the really good news is that once we have figured what the real cause of PMS in women is, we know how to cure the problem**. Read on to find out what the cure is and how to make it work for YOU.

The Natural Hormones Dilemma – Why Doctors Get Confused

It might be hard to believe, but most doctors are indeed confused about natural hormones and especially, progesterone. I was too at one time. Most doctors think a prescription drug called Provera® is the same thing as progesterone. It is not. Provera® is very different chemically.

The reason for this confusion is that we were taught in medical school that Provera® was progesterone. Generations of doctors have believed this and have no clue that Provera® is not progesterone. Furthermore, there is a progesterone-like (but again, not exactly progesterone) drug in birth control pills that doctors confuse with progesterone as well.

Well, here is why. This progesterone "look-alike" is actually a man-made product called Provera®. Provera® happens to be a so-called "progestin" that acts and has characteristics similar to progesterone, but it is NOT progesterone.

The drug company that manufactures Provera® actually takes the natural progesterone molecule and then ALTERS it by adding another chemical group to it. This chemical is another long chemical chain that when added to the base becomes the generic name: medroxy-progesterone. <u>PROVERA® IS **NOT** PROGESTERONE</u>.

All these classes of altered progesterone-like drugs are called progestins. This means that these progesterone look-alike drugs seem to resemble progesterone EXCEPT for some significant chemical alterations which exert their effects on the human body. True, they do have some progesterone like effects BUT at the same time they have enormous number of dangerous side effects.

Side effects of Provera® and other progestins in general were widely publicized in the renowned Women's Health Initiative study a few years ago that have blown the doors off of hormone replacement therapy. I have included a detailed description of this topic in my free report called *"What Nobody Told Women About Hormone Replacement Therapy"*.

The bottom line is that Provera ® and progestins have nasty side effects that include migraine headaches and cancer, just to name a few. The reason why this happens, in my observation, is that <u>these drugs poison the body's production of natural progesterone</u>, thus causing the deficiency of REAL progesterone and a relative imbalance of estrogen excess.

So, naturally comes a question - why do drug companies manufacture drugs that can potentially harm people? The existing patent laws are to blame. In this country and in most others, you cannot patent something that is already found in nature or is already natural. Therefore, in order to patent something, you HAVE to chemically

change it into a non-natural substance. It is THAT simple.

This way, a drug company can then get a patent on this chemical and protect its costly research, development and testing investment in this drug. The reason why drug companies have to chemically alter progesterone into an artificial drug is because of the way that the patent laws are formulated. They just don't have a choice.

However, the problem is that once you alter a natural chemical found in the body into some other chemical that is "foreign" to the organism, that's when all of the side effects come into play.

A good example to show you how just a tiny alteration of a natural hormone can affect the body is the difference between estrogen and testosterone. These are both natural substances found in all humans, men and women. The only differences are the relative amounts of each, with women having a lot of estrogen and a little bit of testosterone and men with the exact opposite.

Looking at the chemical structures of estrogen and testosterone, they seem to be very similar. In fact, the only difference between these two hormones is a single double bond in one of the carbon rings.

Without having to go into complex and boring details from organic chemistry, I will say that the only difference between estrogen and testosterone is a single electron on an atomic level. It's that small and seemingly insignificant difference that separates the two main hormones that make a woman – a woman and a man – a man. Pretty impressive, isn't it?

If a single electron can thus produce the massive physiologic differences between men and women, imagine what an entire, long artificial chemical additive can do to an existing hormone! The side effects of these artificially altered hormones created to satisfy the requirements of the patent laws are tremendous and self-evident.

On the other hand, **natural hormones** (also called **bio-identical hormones**), like progesterone do not have these side effects and never will. The only effects that a natural product like progesterone can affect are those that are dose-related and well known to human physiology. The reason is because in the case of NATURAL progesterone nothing chemically "foreign" is being introduced to the organism.

Of course, if you give someone a lot of progesterone, this will exert more progesterone effects than if you give a small amount of progesterone. It is so simple. These effects are well known and understood.

In fact, a "toxic" dose of progesterone is found in the human condition called - pregnancy!

The amount of the same natural progesterone that I supplement to my female patients is nowhere near the amounts of progesterone circulating in a pregnant woman's body. Thus, unless the FDA and other countries' drug regulators begin labeling pregnancy as a dangerous condition, then we are extremely safe in administering natural progesterone to women.

The Wild Yam Goose Chase

There is a whole industry out there claiming that taking derivatives of wild yams will supplement the body with progesterone. A progesterone precursor, diosgenin, is found in abundance in wild yams. Claims from numerous dietary supplement manufacturers state that the diosgenin found in their yams can supplement the body with progesterone and offer many of the claims that bio-identical progesterone can produce. Well, is that true?

"There is no evidence that the human body converts diosgenin (found in Mexican Wild Yam) to hormones", says Dr. David Zava (PhD in Bio Endocrinology whose focus has been progesterone and estrogen receptor activity) is the Laboratory Director of Aeron Life Cycles - one the foremost hormone testing facilities in the world.

Dr. Zava has tested progesterone levels for many thousands of women and responded with the following: "In response to your question about wild yam steroids - do they convert into progesterone? The answer is NO, there are no enzymes in the human body that will convert diosgenin, the active component of wild yams, into progesterone."

Don't waste your money on the "yam" supplements. They simply just don't work.

THE CURE: How To SUCCESSFULLY Treat PMS

Before I begin, many of you are so motivated that you just read the table of contents and skip immediately to this section and start reading from here.

Because there is quite a bit of background building up to this section, I recommend you start from the beginning. The first 25 pages are relatively easy to read and should only take about 30 minutes of your time. Or you can start here, but do go back later and read from the beginning.

WAIT!

Even if you read nothing else on this page – **I urge you to at least carefully go over the critical information found below** - it's that important!

The Following Information Is

VITALLY IMPORTANT TO YOUR HEALTH

You may be anxious about **"hormones"** – many people are. We've heard so much sensationalized news lately about hormone abuse, it's sometimes difficult to separate **fact from fiction**.

Here's the straight story:

- **PMS is largely caused by a sex hormone deficiency**, though other factors can also play a role.

- **Birth control pills and standard hormone replacement therapy (HRT) are not natural.** They contain chemical "mimics" that only approximate your natural hormones. These mimics are not only **harmful to your body**, but actually cause you to stop making your own NATURAL sex hormones.

- We **make PMS go away** by replenishing deficiencies in your **natural** hormone levels.

- **We use only natural, bio-identical hormones** to replace the deficient hormones your body is lacking.

- Bio-identical hormones are **VERY DIFFERENT** from the hormones you read about in the newspaper. The **prescription hormones** you may have taken in the past (either as birth control pills or HRT) **are NOT NATURAL**.

- **Synthetic hormones are foreign chemicals, acting as poisons.** They shut down your ovaries. They do cause cancer as well as many other health problems.

- However, **BIO-IDENTICAL HORMONES ARE TOTALLY NATURAL!** They are EXACTLY THE SAME as the hormones produced in your own body. **They are absolutely safe** and cannot harm you. They do not cause or contribute to cancer.

- **Mother Nature** would never make a harmful natural hormone. If natural or bio-identical hormones *were* harmful, why don't we see cancers and other health problems in 25 year olds, when hormone production peaks? We don't.

- People get health problems when they take **synthetic, chemically altered hormones that interfere with the body's production of natural hormones**, or when their natural hormone levels decline.

Mainstream Medicine Fails

There is the mainstream medicine method of treating depression which is addressing the symptoms only, and then there is my way – which is **the curative, preventative way**.

First, you should be thoroughly familiar with the mainstream method. If you have downloaded this e-book, then chances are you have already tried virtually every anti-depressant medication known. These include: Effexor, Zoloft, Lexapro, Celexa, Paxil, Elavil, Zyban, and Desyrel.

Recently, one of the drug companies has introduced a new birth control pill called YAZ. They are advertising this Pill as a treatment for PMS (or PMDD as they call it.)

The irony here is that birth control pills (BCP's) are perhaps the biggest single cause of PMS. Yet here this drug company is introducing a BCP to help correct a condition that was caused by a BCP! What a paradox!

Don't believe them. YAZ is not what you should be taking for PMS.

In 2003, estimated sales of antidepressants worldwide were nearly $20 billion (that's TWENTY billion US dollars). One brand alone, Zoloft, accounted for $3.4 billion of that and is the tenth best selling drug in the world. (Source: IMS World Review, 2004.)

Antidepressant sales increase at an annual rate of nearly 10% a year and by 2007 should be approaching nearly THIRTY billion US dollars.

The drug companies have found a partial short term solution to the problem, and have developed these drugs to accommodate a desperate population. Many PMS sufferers do not mind (or have no other choice) paying for something that they are told might help their PMS.

Virtually all of the major drug companies now have their own proprietary antidepressant drug out on the market and they want you to take their version. They have a lot of money invested in these products. It costs hundreds of millions of dollars to research, develop, and pass it through the FDA study process before they get FDA approval to take it to market.

The last thing a drug company needs is to find out that somebody out there has found a cure to the problem that they are making billions off of. Two bad things happen to the drug company at that point:

a) Sales of prescription antidepressant medications will plummet.
b) They just lost several hundred million dollars in development costs.

Therefore, the big drug companies, in partnership with the FDA, will do everything possible to shut down any "natural" source or cure for ANY medical condition that they have invested their money in because natural cures are bad for their business. This also happens to include PMS.

And this means that YOU, the PMS sufferer, will be intentionally denied information and access to any natural, non-prescription or curative product that will make the big drug companies' drugs obsolete.

I will spare you the detailed discussion of these medications. Most of you have already taken one or more of these medications already.

If these medications had worked so well, you would not be reading this book right now. So, assuming that this is correct, then you are ready for the definitive cure for your PMS. I say "definitive" because about 80% of people that I treat are indeed cured by this method.

Why only 80%? Why not 100%?

As with any complicated medical problem we are not always correct in our diagnosis or complete understanding of the underlying disease process. Perhaps the other 20% have some other variation of PMS that we are labeling a hormonal condition but is actually something quite different? And a certain percentage of these people just don't respond as well as we would like to our usual hormone treatment.

If either the progesterone deficiency theory or the estrogen excess withdrawal theory is correct, then the supplementation of progesterone will almost always correct the condition.

This is why curing PMS is so simple and easy – all we do is just add back to women enough progesterone to correct the deficiency in progesterone

This is also why it is 100% natural. Progesterone that is manufactured to exactly match the chemical structure of the real hormone that circulates throughout your body is called **bio-identical**. This is a **natural substance** that every one of us has because our bodies manufacture it on a daily basis.

Please note that I will use the terms "bio-identical hormone" and "natural hormone" interchangeably. They mean exactly the same thing.

To supplement someone with more progesterone that is bio-identical is to do so utilizing an entirely natural approach. All we are doing is supplying in enough quantity to satisfy what the body truly needs to function better.

The results are so striking and occur so quickly that it is gratifying to watch the results.

Women get a little more complicated because we have to deal with the menstrual cycle and get the timing just right within the cycle. Menstruating females ideally will be taking progesterone immediately after ovulation has occurred.

Thus menstruating women should take progesterone supplementation during days 15 -28 (or 30) of their cycle. It may take a couple of cycles or so for PMS (and other gynecological problems) to go away.

A menstruating woman could theoretically take progesterone every day, but this is not usually done when a woman is trying to get pregnant. There is no harm in taking progesterone every day for a menstruating woman, however.

Specifically, progesterone taken during the first half of the menstrual cycle tends to decrease the production of mucous secreted by the uterus. Mucous helps the sperm swim toward the awaiting egg during ovulation.

Also progesterone taken in high dosages can actually suppress ovulation. (This is why pregnant women don't ovulate. – Think about that situation!). But we have many menstruating women taking progesterone on a daily basis for differing reasons. See the comments when I go over the dosage requirements later in this book.

Independent of PMS, for those women who are actively trying to get pregnant, we routinely add progesterone in the second half of the cycle to encourage fertilized egg implantation. Progesterone also prevents or lowers the incidence of miscarriage in the early portion of pregnancy.

Therefore progesterone is quite safe to take for any woman whether they want to get pregnant or not.

Nevertheless, as a matter of routine, we do not usually start out taking progesterone in the first half of your cycle if you are still having periods.

For post-menopausal women, it is much simpler. Take progesterone every single day. No worries, no stress. Very simple. Results come quickly.

What if you are peri-menopausal?

For those of you who do not fall into the traditional classifications of having regular periods (normal menstruating women) and those having no periods (post menopausal) many of you will fall into the "peri-menopausal" group of being in between.

The peri-menopausal woman is typically in her early to late 40's. She is still having periods, but becoming more irregular. The periods can either get lighter and shorter or longer and heavier.

Those peri-menopausal women whose periods are getting longer and heavier typically have uterine fibroids and have been told they may need a hysterectomy. Many have already had a hysterectomy.

For purposes of discussing PMS treatment with progesterone, we separate out those who desire to get pregnant from those who do not. Peri-menopausal women, by definition are pretty much out of the pregnancy running.

So we treat peri-menopausal women as a post-menopausal woman when it comes to hormone replacement with natural progesterone. Alternatively, if you are 37 years old, still cycling normally, but no longer desire to get pregnant, you can take your progesterone supplementation just like the post-menopausal women. There are certain advantages to this schedule as you will see later when we start talking about dosing schedules.

Once the hysterectomy issue comes up, then we get into new categories: those who had a hysterectomy and kept the ovaries and those whose ovaries were removed with the hysterectomy.

Frankly, it doesn't matter whether you have had a hysterectomy or not. Your hormones are still circulating around and every cell in your body is still being affected by them, whether you have a uterus or not.

If your ovaries have been removed, then you discovered a condition called "surgical menopause". This means that while you were still recovering in the hospital following your surgery, you felt immediate menopausal symptoms of hot flashes and night sweats. Because of the sudden shock to your body, this was an intense condition and is likely still troubling you.

I do not intend to go into any detail about menopausal symptoms. We will save that for future topics, but for now as far as progesterone supplementation is concerned, your body is doubly short of progesterone.

Your ovaries are the primary manufacturer of your progesterone and estrogen. When the ovaries were removed your body went into hormone shock. But your body's cells still need those hormones.

The good news is that your adrenal glands can manufacture hormones including progesterone and estrogen. The bad news is that they can't put out the same quantities that your ovaries could make.

The bottom line on natural progesterone supplementation for those of you with hysterectomies, with or without ovarian removal, is that you are now out of the pregnancy class and into the menopausal class. This means you take progesterone supplements every day.

What if you are taking birth control pills?

There is one major step that women **must** do before we start correcting any progesterone deficiency – and that is to **stop taking any birth control pills immediately.** I cannot stress how important it is to discontinue oral contraceptives.

If you do not stop taking birth control pills, then it does not matter what we do, or how much progesterone we give you, you will not get better. Find another method of birth control, just get off the pills. This is not a suggestion, it is mandatory. **Birth control pills are a MAJOR reason why you are getting PMS.**

Stopping birth control pills is not just limited to the oral pills. The same toxic synthetic, chemically altered hormones are also found in birth control patches (Ortho-Evra) and implants like Norplant as well as IUD's and must be removed, as well.

Synthetic hormone replacement drugs like PremPro must also be discontinued. There is more discussion on PremPro later, but this drug gets included in the same category as birth control pills as it is virtually identical to them.

In a nutshell, the reason why birth control pills are so bad for you is because they poison and shut down the body's production of natural progesterone by the ovaries. They also saturate the bloodstream with extra estrogen, giving the worst case scenario of excessive estrogen and insufficient progesterone at the same time.

Please refer to my Special Report, *What Nobody Told Women About Birth Control Pills* for more detailed information on birth control pills and how they have poisoned women across the world.

More to Come:

Following this chapter is a section on Neptune Krill Oil – Nature's Remedy from the Sea. This describes the synergistic effect with natural progesterone that omega-3 fish oil can have on eliminating PMS.

After the Neptune Krill Oil chapter, is a description of a very special type of magnesium supplementation. When added with natural progesterone and Neptune Krill Oil, greatly enhances the cure rate for PMS.

Now, read on for more details on dosages and exactly what to do and where to get it.

Neptune Krill Oil – Nature's Remedy from the Sea

Neptune Krill Oil (NKO) is a remarkable new product that features a natural turbo-charged omega-3 fish oil. One particular type of Krill oil called Neptune Krill Oil has specially integrated omega-3 essential fatty acids – EPA and DHA - that are three times more easily absorbed by the body.

The resulting product is a like a supercharged fish oil that one of the most powerful anti-oxidants on the planet and a very potent anti-inflammatory agent. Yet it is entirely natural, contains no dangerous heavy metals or pesticides and has no fishy aftertaste.

What is unique about Neptune Krill Oil is two-fold: location of where the krill comes from and the process by which it is formulated.

Krill are small shrimp like crustaceans that inhabit the oceans in very cold, deep water off of Antarctica. They are a major food supply for whales, squid, fish and seals. Krill are also found near the Arctic, as well, but they are not as pure as the Antarctic variety.

Neptune is a unique formulation keeping the purity of the krill intact while adding a powerful anti-oxidant to an already potent, naturally occurring substance. It is clearly superior to "generic" brands.

The omega-3 fatty acids in Neptune Krill Oil are exclusively EPA and DHA, come in the form of phospholipids contrary to all other marine oils where the fatty acids are in a triglyceride form. What this means is that the NKO is significantly more bioavailable than fish oil because it allows for direct absorption of EPA and DHA across cell membranes.

The ratio is about 3 to 1, with NKO being absorbed three times faster than traditional fish oil. It passes through the stomach and small intestine so fast that the chance for a fishy aftertaste or reflux is virtually eliminated.

Antioxidant Benefits of Neptune Krill Oil

What makes Neptune Krill Oil so beneficial? It has already been measured to be a very powerful anti-oxidant. Using the Oxygen Radical Absorbance Capacity (ORAC) studies which measure the strength of antioxidant power, NKO has a value 300 times higher than vitamin E and 35 times more potent than Coenzyme Q10. NKO is 47 times more potent as an anti-oxidant than standard fish oil.

Anti-inflammatory Benefits of Neptune Krill Oil

A study showed that Neptune Krill Oil can significantly reduce inflammation by lowering C-reactive protein (CRP) by 30.9% after taking 300mg/day for a period of 30 days. C-reactive protein is one of the most important markers of inflammation measured in blood studies.

Neptune Krill Oil and PMS

A study performed at the University of Montreal and published in the May, 2003 issue of the Alternative Medicine Review, demonstrated a statistically significant improvement in PMS symptoms as measured by a Self-Assessment Questionnaire for the American College of Obstetricians and Gynecologists (ACOG) diagnostic criteria for PMS.

Seventy women took Neptune Krill Oil for 45 days, 90 days or three cycles and demonstrated improvement versus baseline groups who simply took fish oil alone.

This same study also revealed a significant reduction in pain medications needed for dysmenorrheal (painful periods) by those women who took NKO.

Neptune Krill Oil is Synergistic with other Treatments

We have found that the combination of natural progesterone with Neptune Krill Oil and multi-chelated magnesium (see next chapter for magnesium discussion) results in the best overall treatment of PMS.

Obviously, the biggest component is the natural progesterone. Bio-identical progesterone alone works pretty well. Then we added the magnesium product which helped even more.

But the addition of the Neptune Krill Oil seems to be the final accomplishment to the treatment triad. We have raised our success rates even higher with the triple combination.

The Secret Mineral that Will Boost the Effectiveness of Your Program and What No Pharmacists Will Tell You about It

So, what's that magic mineral that makes the sex hormone supplementation program of treating PMS even more effective and what's so secret about it? Well, believe it or not, it's good old **magnesium**. Why? The importance of magnesium for the human body cannot be underestimated. Magnesium is used in over two hundred chemical reactions in a human body.

What's The Secret? Take This and Get an Even Better Response

Magnesium can act synergistically with progesterone to help suppress PMS. There have been two fairly good studies showing that women tend to be deficient in ionized magnesium. One study quantified that 45% of women were low in magnesium.

Keep in mind that about a fourth of the general population is also deficient in magnesium. So there appears to be a higher incidence of magnesium deficiency in women with PMS.

Our clinic has noticed that if you combine magnesium with progesterone supplementation, PMS resolves more quickly than just taking the progesterone alone.

Therefore, we always recommend taking magnesium. But the magnesium has to be a special type that is a little harder to find and that is precisely the "secret" part. There is somewhat of a long explanation to this as people just assume that "magnesium is just magnesium".

Not so.

Please bear with me as it is rather important to explain why getting the right type of magnesium is necessary if we want magnesium to help and give our progesterone supplementation a boost in effectiveness.

Magnesium taken in the form of magnesium oxide is the most common preparation on store and pharmacy shelves. There is a reason for that: It is cheaper to manufacture and comes in a high quantity for the size of the pill.

The problem with magnesium oxide is that it is absorbed and filtered from the body in about an hour. If you try to take it more often, you get diarrhea – not a pleasant long term solution.

So we recommend taking magnesium in the form of a compound that ends with an "ate". Chemical compounds that end in an "ate" are called "chelates".

Chelates are nature's way of neutralizing chemically charged molecules. Magnesium, all by itself, is a mineral that carries an electric charge. It is kind of like a battery. But your body does not like electrically charged substances without some insulation.

So magnesium chelates act as insulators by binding up a molecule that carries that exact opposite electric charge of magnesium. Place the magnesium with the chelate and presto, you have a neutral, zero charged chemical complex.

A magnesium chelate vastly improves the bodies ability to absorb and take it up for immediate use in the myriad of physiological reactions where it is required.

The following are all examples of magnesium chelates.

- Magnesium aspartate,
- Magnesium gluconate,
- Magnesium glycinate,
- Magnesium stearate,
- And/or magnesium citrate

These are the best magnesium supplements to take because they absorb the best, last longer inside the body and are cleared more slowly by the kidneys.

However, each of the magnesium chelate compounds will last inside the body for a particular time, like 2 hours to 8 hours. They all have different "peaks" and "valleys" in terms of how much magnesium is released inside the body.

The idea is to find a magnesium supplement that combines multiple chelates into one pill so your body can have continuous high magnesium coverage for up to eight hours. Then you take this ideal magnesium pill just three times a day and you are covered with sufficient magnesium.

We found one magnesium product that actually contains not one, but three of the above magnesium chelates. This will be described for you in the "How Do We Get These Treatments" chapter later in this book. I will also tell you how you can get your own magnesium chelate formula as one of your treatment options.

THE PLAN: Exact Dosages and Administration

Print this section out and read it carefully.

Be sure and read every word in this section, even in those sections that you don't think apply to you because some of the comments apply to all women, regardless of category.

After years of practice, a lot of trial and error, and incredible feedback from my early patients who were not afraid of some experimentation, we have finally figured out the best overall doses of progesterone to give.

For Menstruating Women:

Be sure and know which category you are in. There is a detailed discussion in the "How Do We Treat PMS" section above describing who is considered to be a menstruating woman and who is not in the category (even if you are still having periods).

The best rule of thumb is that if you are having periods and are of child bearing age and still desire (or would not mind) having any more children, then you are considered to be in the menstruating woman category.

The age group for this category begins with young girls experiencing their very first periods up to women approaching age 40. We have successfully treated girls as young as 13 who were going through menarche, which is the medical term given for having your very first periods.

1. The best dose to give a menstruating woman is 50 mg of bio-identical or natural progesterone given twice daily from days 15 through 28 (or day 30 or the last day of the cycle before menstruation starts).

2. In addition to the progesterone recommended dosage, to make this treatment plan work even better, take 100 mg of long-acting magnesium, three times a day.

3. Neptune Krill Oil: Take one gel cap twice daily.

If you are currently taking birth control pills, do not start taking the bio-identical progesterone until you finish out your last round of birth control pills. In other words, regardless of where you are on the birth control pack, finish all 28 pills (or 21 if your pack comes this way) and wait for your menstrual period to start as usual. Then you can throw away your remaining oral contraceptives forever.

A special note on young girls and teenagers who are experiencing terrible periods and have PMS: Almost all of them have been placed on birth control pills by mainstream medicine and this just worsens the PMS.

So your daughters who are caught in this situation need to get off the pill as described in the preceding paragraph.

Remember that day one of your cycle is the first day of bleeding with your period. So after you finish your birth control pills for the prior month, then begin with the progesterone on day 15 of the following month. Then continue to take as instructed above – for days 15 through 28 (or 30, or the last day before your period starts).

If you are not taking oral contraceptives currently, you can just start taking the progesterone the next time your day 15 comes up. Timing is very important, so you don't want to jump the gun and start taking these bio-identical progesterone hormones too soon or too late.

For Non-Menstruating *or* Post Menopausal Women *or* Peri-Menopausal *or* Women with Hysterectomies:

This category is for everybody else. For classification purposes we will call this giant category the "Post-Menopausal Category". There will be discussion below on post-menopausal dosage changes and all of the women who are peri-menopausal and those with hysterectomies will be considered to be part of this post-menopausal group.

We can even include those of you who are not yet peri-menopausal, are somewhere around your late 30's and desire no more children.

This category is much simpler because we don't have to count days anymore.

1. The best dose to give a non-menstruating woman is 50 mg given twice daily, every day. Medications in a pill or capsule form by mouth are best.

2. In addition to the progesterone recommended dosage, to make this treatment plan work even better, take 100 mg of long-acting magnesium, three times a day.

3. Neptune Krill Oil: Take one gel cap twice daily.

There is no need to have a periodic week off (literally). Natural progesterone is so safe that you can take it every day, forever.

At the recommended dosages your periods, if any, are not likely to change much. If they do change, they will get lighter, shorter or disappear altogether. This is not a problem and we have never had any woman complain about lighter, shorter or no periods.

Range of Dosages:

Smaller doses are helpful, but these dosages are usually not curative. Higher doses are safe as well, but we don't want to start out too high. This is the Goldilocks principle – not too small, not too large, but just right.

We can easily give double those recommended amounts and be extremely safe. Don't forget that during pregnancy there is four times more progesterone circulating around in a woman's body than the dosage that we are administering to cure PMS.

Partial Response?

What if you tried taking the recommended dosage of 50 mg twice a day for two or three months and your PMS is less frequent and/or less intense, but still present? Simple – just increase the dose.

The formula is to incrementally add 50 mg of progesterone every couple of months until the PMS is gone - up to a maximum daily dose of 200 mg/day.

So, if you are one of those women who've been taking progesterone for two or three months and have received a "partial response", here is what you should do:

Beginning the following month, start adding an additional 50 mg of progesterone to your daily dose. So your next increment would be 50 mg in the morning and 100 mg in the evening on days 15 -28 for menstruating women and daily for post-menopausal women (everybody else). Try that for two months and see what happens.

After two more months have passed, if the PMS is improving, but still not gone completely, you may increase the dose again. Add an additional 50 mg of progesterone. So now it would be up to 100 mg two times a day (morning and evening). Again, progesterone should be taken on days 15-28 of your cycle for menstruating women and every day if you are post menopausal.

When we get to this level, I usually put menstruating women on 50 mg, just once a day, on days 1 – 14 as well. To clarify, menstruating women will take 50 mg of progesterone on days 1- 14 and then 100 mg of progesterone, two times daily, during days 15 – 28. Keep in mind that it takes about 6 months of partial responses to get to this level. Most menstruating women never need to worry about this.

For post-menopausal women and everyone else who is not in the menstruating woman category, the maximum dose is 100 mg two times a day taken every day.

Breast Fullness:

Some women will experience breast fullness or soreness when they start taking progesterone. This is especially true for the higher dosages. Don't worry, this is a normal response and should go away in a few weeks or sooner.

If the breast fullness is just too painful and/or there are other symptoms like ankle swelling (water retention) or worsening of pre-existing PMS symptoms, then it could be because we started the progesterone dose too high.

If this is the case, then it could be because your body is so deficient in progesterone that our starting dose was too high and your body actually converted some of it into estrogen, which worsens the situation.

If this happens, then lower the progesterone to just 50 mg taken only in the evening. Try this for a couple of months. Then you can work up from there depending on the response of your PMS.

The goal is to find the smallest dose that will make your PMS go away.

What If Your PMS Gets Worse Temporarily?

Just like the breast fullness discussion above, some women are so deficient in progesterone that they actually get worsening of the PMS when starting this dosage regimen. If that happens, just back off to one 50 mg progesterone capsule in the evening.

Then you will need to let your body adapt to the new amounts of progesterone circulating around. You will likely have to increase the dosages over time to make your PMS go away completely.

Other Medications:

Simplicity is always best. If you are taking any other medications, for any other reason, continue to take them as usual. The addition of progesterone should not affect any other prescription or non-prescription medication you are currently taking. (Except for birth control pills. You will need to get off of those as outlined above.)

The reason why I don't recommend changing any of your medications is simply based on the fact that we don't want to change more than one variable at a time. As a general rule, the body does not like change, so we keep it simple by just adding or subtracting one component at a time.

Premarin® vs. PremPro®

If you are currently taking hormone replacement therapy for hot flashes or night sweats in the form of Premarin® or other similar estrogens, you should stay on them. There is no need to discontinue any other hormone (unless it contains the synthetic Provera® component like PremPro®). This is the same artificial progestin found in birth control pills.

If you are taking PremPro®, then this will need to be changed to just Premarin® without the "Pro". But just like the women on birth control pills, you must get off the PremPro®. Otherwise, your PMS will not go away.

Because we are dealing with prescriptions here, you will need your doctor's cooperation on this. However, with all the bad press on PremPro®, I doubt any doctor will have a problem changing out PremPro® back to just Premarin®.

IUD's and Implants

If you are on any IUD's with medication in them or an implant like Norplant, those need to be removed. These are essentially identical to birth control pills in their effects. You will not get better until these are removed.

Some IUD's do not have any medication embedded within them. These are the old fashioned copper IUD's. If this is what you have, then they can stay.

Anti-Depressants:

As much as I dislike anti-depressants, if you are already on them (most women with PMS are already taking them, unfortunately), continue to take them as before. Go ahead and start the progesterone as instructed as we change nothing else on your medication regimen.

Over time, as your PMS disappears and never returns, *then* you can discontinue the anti-depressants. Again, let your doctor manage the discontinuation process for these drugs, as many of them need to be slowly weaned off of, rather than abruptly stopped.   Your doctor should be happy to do this for you as you no longer need these drugs anymore.

Special Situations:

If you follow my program strictly, your PMS should go away after a couple of cycles, or about 60 days. Hence, my reference to getting cured in 60 days on my website. Don't be surprised, however, if you should experience occasional breakthrough PMS symptoms, possibly once or twice a year.

For some reason, we do come across some women whose PMS will breakthrough, despite adhering pretty well to my program. If this happens, do NOT stop the program. Continue taking the progesterone under my recommendations. Do not lose the faith! – and stay with the program.

You will notice, that if you do have "breakthrough" PMS symptoms, that it is milder and shorter than what you experienced before. Not everyone will get another round of PMS but occasionally some patients do.

Timing Matters!

Sometimes we *can* explain why someone might get breakthrough PMS. Timing matters! When the recommendation says to begin on day 15, I mean you start taking the progesterone on day 15, not day 16. Starting one day late makes a difference. I have observed mild PMS symptoms when women are only one or two days behind schedule.

Keep a close record of your menstrual calendar. Day one is the first day of bleeding. Day 15 is exactly two weeks later. Don't miss it. If you cannot remember, it is better strategy to take your progesterone a day early rather than a day too late. There is no such thing as too much progesterone. There is definitely such a thing as insufficient progesterone, however.

Your Cycle and How it Responds to Stress

Another observation is that your menstrual cycle is vulnerable to outside stimuli that can change the cycle. For example, excessive stress, infections and even things like travel (especially airplane and particularly when crossing several time zones at once). Going to the mountains with an elevation in altitude can alter the menstrual cycle.

Another example is every winter we have an upsurge in PMS. The cold weather does not help. Catching the flu almost always triggers PMS no matter how good you are with the treatment program.

One interesting observation we have made is the relationship of travel with PMS. For some reason there is a tendency to get some PMS symptoms about three or four days after traveling, especially by air. The airport experience apparently has gotten so stressful that it must be significantly affecting the body.

My theory on why a stressful situation results in PMS a few days later concerns the body's ability to contain stress. Stress is a real physiologic condition where your adrenal glands produce adrenaline during the acute hyper stress phase.

But when the stressful event fades away, i.e. you finished your travel or getting over the flu, your body stops making adrenaline and starts to relax. Boom! That is when you get the symptoms.

Why is this? The theory is because your body is probably deficient in cortisol, which is another hormone your adrenal gland makes that circulates around longer and is slower acting in response to stress.

Most women that I have treated have been so stressed out over a couple of decades that their adrenal glands are worn out and just quit making cortisol hormones to a sufficient level that protects the body from longer term stress.

Effect of Prescription Medications on PMS

Prescription medications, especially steroids and even some antibiotics can lengthen, but more likely shorten the cycle. Finally, I have seen injected steroids, like pain shots or epidural steroid injections, which have caused premature menstrual periods.

Anything that changes your menstrual cycle also changes the hormones that affect it. Therefore, possible breakthrough PMS symptoms can occur in each of the above scenarios. The best you can do is just to follow your calendar as best as you can. If there is a change in the cycle, then react accordingly and start the progesterone on the **new** day 15.

Breakthrough PMS may occur anyway, but if you can minimize the external stimuli that keep affecting your cycle, it should iron out in a couple of months. Whatever you do, do not stop the program!

Following the program means that you will be taking bio-identical progesterone for the rest of your life. This is the intention and not a problem. The progesterone that you are about to take is not addictive in any way. You can get off any time. Your body will wash out of the added natural progesterone in just a few days.

But your body will soon revert back to its old ways of being deficient in progesterone. Eventually, your condition will revert back to the old days of cyclic PMS and other problems, just like it was before you started taking progesterone supplementation. This is just simple physiology at work.

Pills vs. Creams:

Another delivery system besides taking medications by mouth is the skin (topical application). The problem with skin administration of progesterone (or any other medication) is the extreme variation in absorption through the skin. The skin varies tremendously in its absorption properties in different parts of the body and even in the identical place during the same day.

The reason why the skin is so variable has to do with temperature, whether the skin sub-surface blood vessels are wide open or mostly closed, the amount of sweat and sweat glands. Furthermore, it is very difficult to apply the same amount of cream consistently from a tube.

There is a great deal of variation of product density within the tube with some portions of the tube being very high concentration and other portions being almost completely taken up by fillers.

This is worsened by the fact that creams are difficult to manufacture from one lot to another with any consistency. Few batches of creams are exactly alike. From a manufacturing perspective, it is extremely difficult to get the same cream mixture and consistency each and every time. A batch made last month may be as much as 20% off from one made today.

I have already done the research on cream absorption. Many cream advocates say that the skin is superior in absorption over oral administration because the liver will remove much of the oral dose but the skin does not have to worry about that.

Yes, the skin does absorb chemicals quite well. But the problem is the predictability of how much your skin will absorb versus a known amount by mouth. Your skin never absorbs the same way twice.

Oral medications, on the other hand, are more predictable in their absorption.

Finally, the FDA has some archaic rules preventing cream manufacturers from making a dense enough cream to really help. As a result, to achieve therapeutic doses from a cream, a woman must literally take a bath in the cream.

This is extremely inconvenient, not to mention quite expensive as you end up spending three or four times what was advertised.

The end result is that topical (via skin) dosages vary all over the map and consistency is virtually impossible to maintain. The body will see wild variations in progesterone coming at it and this may actually worsen the condition. In contrast, oral administration is easy, convenient, predictable and safe.

Pills are much easier to take, more convenient to use, and easier to manufacture in a consistent fashion. As a result, blood levels of progesterone are more consistent and predictable.

If a particular oral dose is not effective or just practically effective, then we just increase the dose until it works. Easy. No guess work. No mess.

THE SOURCES: Finding The Products – Quickly and Easily

Obtaining the above recommended dosages of progesterone can be done in a variety of ways. They vary in how much you wish to pay and what kind of extra services you desire.

OPTION 1:

Perhaps the best and most thorough means of getting the right treatment and dosages of progesterone is to go to one of the boutique medical clinics that some of my more enterprising colleagues have established. These clinics advertise themselves as natural medicine, natural hormones, women's health, anti-aging or some similar marketing measures.

You may have seen some advertising for these clinics on billboards or in your local suburban home type of magazines that target high income demographic groups or a magazine in the seat pocket of an airline seat. These boutique practices do not accept insurance but gladly accept your credit card in the amounts near $4000 just to get in the door.

Of course, for your $4000, you get to sip tea from fine china in the reception area, sit on fine furniture on the oriental rugs placed on top of hardwood floors and gaze at some really nice artwork on the walls.

The doctors and staff treat you like royalty and you have a pleasant experience. At the end of the day, you will have the world's most expensive progesterone dosage program, but it works.

Here is the link to perhaps the finest boutique clinic in America that can do this: www.hotzehwc.com

OPTION 2:

You can fly down and come to my clinic and we will do a complete consultation and physical examination. Simply send an email to info@PMScure.com or call 281-962-4264 and we will be more than happy to see you in the clinic.

Compared to Option 1 above, my office does not have the fine china, the oriental rugs or the nice artwork. But by the time you finished the initial visit and all of the myriad items that go with it, you would still be paying nearly $2000 from your credit card and insurance is not accepted. Please note that this covers only the doctor visit portion. You still have to obtain your supply of progesterone elsewhere.

Obviously our clinic accountant would love for you to come on down to Houston and visit us. But there are more practical methods than this.

My goal is to spread the word on proper treatment of PMS to as many women worldwide as possible. Keeping this information and treatment reserved exclusive to only the very wealthy is not my idea of accomplishing this.

However, some people just enjoy spending money and we will accept it, but there are better options.

OPTION 3:

Another option is to see if your regular doctor would be willing to write a prescription for the progesterone dosages noted above. Very few doctors on the planet know how to manage bio-identical hormones, particularly when it comes to PMS.

My observation is that most mainstream medical doctors have a) never heard of bio-identical progesterone and would try to write you a prescription for Provera® instead, or b) lecture you on his perception of the "danger" of using natural hormones instead of his comfort zone of prescription drugs created by big drug companies with their myriad of side effects.

Most people do have a good relationship with their doctor. After all, anyone with PMS has likely visited their doctor on numerous occasions and had a number of phone calls as well.

The problem is even if your doctor writes out a prescription for bio-identical progesterone in the recommended dosages, you still have to buy it from a compounding pharmacist. That gets expensive.

Compounding pharmacies, by definition, create just one prescription at a time for a specified patient. They make it by hand with no automation and it is slow, tedious and very expensive. Before my clinic found an alternate means of obtaining bio-identical progesterone, I had no choice but to work with compounding pharmacies in my area.

A typical compounding pharmacy will charge a minimum of one US dollar per capsule, regardless of the dose or even the drug they put in it. The manual labor to make it overwhelms all other costs. So a prescription for 60 capsules in a bottle runs a minimum of US$60.

I remember only a couple of years ago when a capsule was "only" 80 cents a capsule – and we thought that was high. I see more and more compounding pharmacies headed towards the US$1.10 - $1.15 per capsule range now with no end in sight.

The pharmacies must be thinking that they have a monopoly on the creation of natural hormones and believe they can raise the price indefinitely until people start complaining about it more. Little do they know about how the marketplace responds to the need for women to have high quality and low cost natural hormones.

Fortunately, we found a better and far less expensive option that enables you to bypass seeing your doctor and you can obtain natural progesterone for a fraction of the cost that you would pay otherwise.

OPTION 4:

A final option, as well as the simplest and least expensive method, is to find a progesterone product that accomplishes all of my criteria: Oral administration, pure quality, easily shipped, convenient to use and inexpensive. We finally found a way around the expensive compounding pharmacy source of natural hormones.

Frankly, we got tired of dealing with the tactics of compounding pharmacies. My patients were facing price increase after price increase, so we started searching around for other options to get them their progesterone.

After a great deal of searching around and research, I have found one progesterone product that satisfies all of the necessary criteria. This is the only non-prescription form of oral progesterone on the planet as far as we can tell.

It can be shipped to you in the exact dose of progesterone (50mg) in capsule form. The really good news is that you can get a month's supply of progesterone (for a menstruating woman) for about

US$15 and you don't need to see a doctor or get a prescription. You can just order it off the internet.

Once we found this supplier, we started ordering it for our own clinic patients. Since we use so much of it ourselves, I investigated this product and had their progesterone tested in a quality control lab for verification that it was:

a) TRUE bio-identical to human progesterone
b) Actually contains 50 mg of progesterone within each capsule.

   It passed in both categories.

You can order it off the manufacturer's website at www.progest50.com .

Another feature I like about option #4 is that it comes in 50 mg capsules. I always work in 50 mg increments when it comes to dosage changes and this makes it very convenient.

We have been very pleased with this supplier. American customers receive their orders in a few days and international orders are received in a week or so.

Shipping charges are not very expensive. For domestic American shipping, it costs about 50 cents a month. For our international customers, it runs about one US dollar per month for shipping. No one has reported back to us about any customs, tariffs or governmental regulation problems – and we have customers in many countries all over the world.

I get e-mails from my international customers wondering if they can get this progesterone product in their home country. So far, we have not heard of any problems with them receiving their orders in any country.

Some further comments on this particular product, Progest 50:

Here is how the $15/month cost is calculated: You have to purchase the "buy 3 get 2 free" offer from the Progest50 internet site. This costs about US$150 for five bottles. Each bottle contains 60 capsules. Assuming that a menstruating woman takes two capsules daily for half the month, each bottle works out to a two month supply. Five bottles then lasts 10 months, or $15/month.

Non-menstruating women taking a daily Progest50 dose would be twice as much or US$30/month.

The bottle also has a lot of legal language that I have to comment on. Keep in mind that the manufacturer is in America and this label is obviously written by a lawyer, not a doctor. Welcome to the legal climate in America.

The instructions on the bottle tell you to take one capsule two times daily. That's fine, but go back to my instructions on dosages and look up what you need to do if there is a partial response. Be sure and print out my chapter on Dosages and Administration.

The label also says it is not for men or for individuals under 18 years. I agree about the men part, but we do have 13 and 14 year old girls taking it as per my recommendations.

It also talks about not taking it if you are trying to get pregnant, already pregnant or nursing. That is lawyer talk – you can ignore that part. We actually encourage this to women who are trying to get pregnant or are already pregnant.

I also recommend it during nursing because a woman who has just delivered a brand new baby will have a significant chance of post-partum depression, not to mention the return of migraine headaches. So we do use it then.

Finally, the label advises you not to take it if you are using various forms of birth control pills or patches. I agree. You should stop all birth control pills in the manner that has been discussed above.

A Word About Those Progesterone Creams

Many of you are already using a progesterone based cream. I get a lot letters asking if you can continue using them.

As already discussed above, progesterone creams are relatively ineffective. Since so many of you who are using them STILL get PMS – that only underscores their failure to help in this situation.

You might believe simply increasing the amount of cream will alleviate your PMS. Sorry – that won't work. Here's why:

- **Dosages:** First, you have no idea what dosages you're using because it requires an enormous amount of cream to reach a therapeutic level. By that time you're literally taking a bath in the stuff - with all of the hassles that scenario conjures up.

- **Potency:** Don't forget about the manufacturing problems we talked about. Cream manufacturers don't tell you about the variability of hormones within different batches, much less within the same tube. Skin absorption also varies widely. While skin does absorb chemicals quite well, it never absorbs the same way twice. On those days when skin absorption isn't quite up to par, you run the very real risk of a breakthrough PMS symptoms.

- **Convenience:** Face it – creams are messy, smelly and don't exactly feel great on the skin either. Which would you rather do: Plaster yourself with viscous gunk – or swallow a convenient pill? (That's an easy choice!)

- **Cost:** Finally, creams multiply the cost three or four fold. The preparation you thought was such a bargain can end up costing you US$80 - $100 per month. Not so cheap anymore – is it?

MAGNESIUM SUPPLEMENTATION

Supplementing with magnesium is important because of the synergistic or additive effects we see when combined with your natural progesterone. Extensive discussion of adding magnesium has already been mentioned above in the "*The Secret Mineral that Will Boost the Effectiveness of Your Program and What No Pharmacist Will Tell You about It*" section.

Magnesium supplements are manufactured in a myriad of formulations and products. The most common magnesium supplement product you will see at any pharmacy or health food store is in the form of magnesium oxide.

I have already discussed magnesium oxide above and how ineffective it is. You need a superior chemically compatible magnesium compound for your body.

My favorite is a combination of magnesium compounds ending in "ates":

- Magnesium aspartate,
- Magnesium gluconate,
- Magnesium glycinate,
- Magnesium stearate,
- And/or magnesium citrate

As a service to our patients, my staff and I did the field work and research to find the very best magnesium product that met the necessary criteria: multiple "ates", high quality, convenient, and inexpensive. There are hundreds, if not thousands of magnesium products out there and we found the very best one we could recommend for you.

It is called Mg-Zyme and manufactured by Biotics Research. Usually, a magnesium product, if it has an "ate" in it will just have one kind. This Mg-Zyme actually has *three*:

- Magnesium aspartate,
- Magnesium gluconate,
- And magnesium glycinate

We actually toured the manufacturing plant. This is where the workers are wearing NASA-like space suits inside the "clean rooms" where the pills are made. It reminded me of the same plant manufacturing quality that the computer chip manufacturers use.

An independent lab has already verified the batch for quality composition.

Mg-Zyme comes in quantity of 100 tablets with each tablet weighing in at 100 mg each. At three times a day dosage, one bottle works out to a little better than a month's supply.

The best part is the price – only US$15 per bottle - or about US$13.50 per month at my recommended dosages.

The only catch is that Biotics Research usually does not sell to the general public. You have to be a patient of one of their approved doctors to buy their products. To enable you to get access to Mg-Zyme, we have set up an account with them, but **when you call you have to tell them that you have been referred to them by Dr. Andrew Jones - otherwise you can't get it**. Also, they may ask for a doctor ID number. Here it is: **05TD5252**.

They can only take orders via telephone using live operators during their business hours (CST, which is GMT-6). Their phone number is 1-800-231-5777 for US customers. Their regular phone number for international calls is
+1 281-344-0909. They can ship anywhere in the world. If you need to look them on the internet, their website address is www.MagnesiumOrder.com .

Neptune Krill Oil Supplementation

Supplementing with Neptune Krill Oil (NKO) is important because of the synergistic or additive effects we see when combined with your natural progesterone. Extensive discussion of adding NKO has already been mentioned above in the *"Neptune Krill Oil – Natures Remedy from the Sea"* section.

There are a number of Neptune Krill Oil preparations on the market. Our favorite, by far, is a form of NKO that not only naturally packages the omega-3 fatty acids into a phospholipid molecule carrier that makes absorption three times better than standard fish oils, but also contains added astaxanthin, a very powerful anti-oxidant.

Neptune Krill Oil is also 47 times more potent as an anti-oxidant than standard fish oil. As you can see, NKO is clearly superior to fish oil. With the addition of natural astaxanthin, which is six times more potent than fish oil, the final product is very effective.

Where to Get Neptune Krill Oil

After doing extensive searching and watching results, my recommendation for the best product on the market can be found by ordering from Rejuvenation Science online at http://KrillOil.PMScure.com . If you click directly on this link, you will be directed to a VIP area for my patients and become entitled to a 10% discount off their retail price.

Rejuvenation Science is clearly the most effective formulation. There are cheaper generics of Neptune Krill Oil out there, but they are less effective.

Recommended Dosage:

The recommended dosage is to take one gel cap twice daily. NKO by itself is insufficient to cure your PMS. You must take it in combination with the progesterone and magnesium.

Levels of Potency

Analyzing the three components taken synergistically to eliminate your PMS there is a hierarchy of potency. Ideally you should take all three (progesterone, Neptune Krill Oil and magnesium chelates) to best enhance the outcome. But if your budget is limited, then you need to know how to prioritize these recommendations.

By far, the bio-identical progesterone is the most important and the most effective in eliminating PMS. So if your budget forces you to choose just one, go with the progesterone.

The next most important is the Neptune Krill Oil and combine with the bio-identical progesterone.

Then follow with the magnesium chelate product and combine with the other two as the best possible treatment recommendation. The combination of progesterone plus NKO plus magnesium in the right doses becomes a triumvirate working in concert with each other to best enhance the elimination of PMS.

Combining the NKO with the magnesium without the progesterone is still not as effective as the natural progesterone alone. So stick with the progesterone at all costs.

Use all three and you will get the best result that way.

Other Supplements

Before I close, let me comment that regardless of your PMS status, that you (and your family – everyone should be taking these) should be taking the following supplements:

- Multivitamins (with large amounts of B vitamins)

- Krill Oil - this is the latest and best version of omega-3 oil
  (source: http://KrillOil.PMScure.com)

- Vitamin C – at least 3000mg per day

- Calcium – at least 1000 – 1500mg per day

- Magnesium chelates – see prior recommendations: 300 mg/day (source: http://MagnesiumOrder.com)

- Folic Acid – 400 mcg/day

- Vitamin E – 400 IU's/day

- Vitamin D - 400 IU's/day

- Probiotics – Primal Defense

- Kefir – 8 – 16 ounces/day

We recommend other supplements in other specialty situations, but that is beyond the scope of this book.

Summary of Recommendations:

1. Progesterone – 50 mg, twice daily (or days 15 – 28 if menstruating) Source: www.Progest50.com

2. Neptune Krill Oil – One gel cap twice daily Source: http://KrillOil.PMScure.com

3. Magnesium Chelates – One tablet, three times a day
   Source: www.MagnesiumOrder.com   Doctor ID: 05TD5252

4. Other Supplements - See above

Summary of Recommendations – At a Glance

For those of you who want to get straight to the recommendations of what to do and where to get it here they are:

Summary of Recommendations:

1. Progesterone – 50 mg, twice daily (or days 15 – 28 if menstruating) Source: www.Progest50.com

2. Neptune Krill Oil – One gel cap twice daily Source: http://KrillOil.PMScure.com

3. Magnesium Chelates – One tablet, three times a day
Source: www.MagnesiumOrder.com   Doctor ID: 05TD5252

4. Other Supplements - See page 54

What to Do if All Else Fails – (The "20%")

This chapter is reserved only for those women who have done EVERYTHING recommended thus far, but still have terrible PMS. Before we go on, let's review the steps you should have gone through before declaring the treatment program a failure:

- Did you take bio-identical progesterone (Progest50) at the 50mg doses twice daily during days 15 – 28 of the month for menstruating women or every day for everyone else?

- If that failed,
  Did you double the dose to 100 mg during the same days?

- If that failed,
  Did you expand the days taken to everyday if you are menstruating?

- If that failed,
  Did you increase the dose to 150mg per day?

- If that failed,
  Did you increase the dose to 200mg per day?

- If that failed,
  Did you take the magnesium chelates as recommended?

- Are you taking the bio-identical progesterone from Progest50 or from some other source? I only trust Progest50. Not Prometrium. Not compounded by someone else. And definitely not a progesterone cream.

- Did you stop birth control pills?

- Did you stop synthetic hormone replacement therapy? (This includes PremPro and all estrogenic drugs).

- Did you remove contraceptive implants or IUD's tainted with synthetic, chemically altered progestins?

Are you taking any other powerful medications that influence hormone levels like:

- Steroids (this includes steroid creams or inhalers)
- Anti-depressant medications
- Blood pressure medications (like beta-blockers, eq. Inderal)
- Psychotropic drugs (Zyprexa, Seroquel, Risperdol)
- Amphetamines (Ritalin, Adderal)
- Sleep aids
- Valium-like drugs

Have you looked at a great website for information: www.DitchThePill.org ?

If you done all of the above, then is officially a treatment failure. It also took several months to get to this point. Now let's discuss this further.

Do You Also Have These Problems?

One observation I have made consistently on the treatment failures is that they tend to have one or more of the following health problems above and beyond PMS. These include:

- Yeast condition
- Irritable bowel syndrome (probably related to yeast)
- Low thyroid
- Chronic Fatigue Syndrome
- Fibromyalgia (probably related to Chronic Fatigue Syndrome)

Stop and Take This On-LineTest

At this point, I want you to stop and take an online test. Go to www.HotzeHWC.com and take their on-line questionnaire. It covers the above topics. Tally up your score and then come back to this chapter when you are finished.

Most of you will score high in one or more of the above categories. Once you have established that, then continue to read on for further explanation and instructions.

Yeast

Yeast is a huge topic all by itself. The terms "yeast" and "Candida" are interchangeable. Candida are simply multiple strains of yeast. There are probably hundreds of Candida strains that comprise yeast. They are all toxic.

Mainstream medicine virtually totally ignores yeast, but it is epidemic and endemic. Almost every woman on the planet has had a "yeast infection" at one time in her life, so women know what yeast is, even if her doctor doesn't.

Yeast is much more than just a vaginal yeast infection. Yeast is actually a type of mold or fungus. Yeast lives just about everywhere except in extreme dry climates. Even so, yeast still lives INSIDE YOU.

Our bodies are colonized with yeast just like our intestines are colonized with bacteria – some friendly, some harmful. If bacteria can live inside our intestines, why can't yeast? They also live in your sinuses, your vagina and sometimes in your skin, toenails, inner ear and any other place in or on your body.

As babies we are exposed and colonized with yeast (remember diaper rash? – that is yeast). Oral thrush in babies is also yeast. How about those ear infections? Mainstream medicine hands out reams of antibiotics and guess what? We get yeast to colonize the ear canals afterwards.

Yeast are everywhere and we can't do anything about it. But when we take antibiotics or steroids, the balance of power between yeast and bacteria changes. Antibiotics indiscriminately kill off beneficial bacteria which results in an overgrowth of yeast.

Dysbiosis and Irritable Bowel Syndrome

Yeast produce toxins that circulate and cause dozens of strange symptoms. Yeast are responsible for "dysbiosis", which is an overgrowth of yeast in the intestines resulting in gas, bloating, abdominal pain, diarrhea that mainstream medicine calls Irritable Bowel Syndrome (IBS).

Unfortunately, mainstream medicine completely misses the boat on how to effectively treat IBS. They have identified the symptoms but haven't figured out what causes it and definitely have no idea how to cure it. They just throw toxic medications at it.

Yeast are also responsible for chronic sinus conditions, ear infections and many allergies. They are almost always present in people who have resistant PMS.

If you wish to learn more on the subject, a couple of good books to read are: *The Yeast Syndrome* and

The Yeast Connection. They are available from Amazon's website at the following links:

http://AmazonYeastSyndrome.pmscure.com and http://AmazonYeastConnection.pmscure.com.

Doctors have no idea how to treat IBS or any other yeast condition acquired outside of a hospital. You will need a yeast-killing antibiotic like Diflucan, Nizoral or Sporonox. Nizoral is the least expensive one and works just as well as the others.

You will need to take one of those yeast killers for a LONG TIME - like 6 months. I personally took Sporonox for 8 months in a row. (I had the same thing you did). Doctors will fall out of their chair when you request a 6 month supply of one of these medications, but I speak from experience.

You will also need to take an anti-yeast drug, called Nystatin, three or four times a day that kills intestinal yeast on contact. Nystatin is not absorbed into the bloodstream and stays strictly inside the intestines.

Another major weapon to use against yeast is a class of dietary supplements called "probiotics". Basically these are the "good" bacteria that you need to colonize your intestines. These are the bacteria that help your digestion process.

They are essential to healthy digestion. Good bacteria, like *lactobacillus* species have a symbiotic relationship with us. In exchange for free room and board inside our intestines, they help us digest our foods. It is a win-win relationship.

Unfortunately that relationship gets altered when we introduce antibiotics or steroids into our bodies. Good bacteria help suppress yeast and bad bacteria that want to set up shop inside you. When antibiotics indiscriminately kill off good bacteria and the bad at the same time, not only does that encourage yeast growth, but it also encourages an overgrowth of bad bacteria.

Primal Defense

In order to keep the body's digestive tract well colonized with good bacteria, we recommend probiotics daily. My favorite probiotic is called Primal Defense. It is manufactured by the Garden of Life people and you can get it from health food stores and Whole Foods Markets.

Work up to 6 Primal Defense tablets/day divided into 2 daily doses on an empty stomach. In other words, take three in the morning when you get up and three at night. Do not start taking 6 tablets when you first start. You slowly work up to that level starting with just one a day for a couple of days. Then go to two, then three, etc., until you reach the total of six.

Kefir

Another great product as an add-on to Primal Defense (not in place of it), is a dairy product called Kefir. It is like yogurt, but several times better. Many gastroenterologists consider it to be the world's most perfect food item. I agree. You just cannot get enough it.

The plain, unflavored version tastes very similar to buttermilk. Many people like it (myself included). If you are not a fan of the unflavored version, try the flavored versions – strawberry, blueberry, vanilla and the like.

Kefir is so mainstream nowadays that many regular grocery stores are starting to carry it. If yours does not, try a health food store.

But don't limit it just for yourself. Your entire family will benefit from the world's most healthy beverage. This also includes your children. (There is even a special line of "kid kefir". The only difference from the adult brand is that it is entirely organic.

Worthless Candida Remedies

Some people describe long holistic yeast (Candida) treatment experiences that involve incredible complex programs from strict diets to "purges". They have usually been on multiple herbal remedies. The diets are impossible to maintain. And nothing has worked.

I have no trouble with diet alterations (reducing the carb intake), or purges, or any of these items. But until you add the yeast killing drugs mentioned above, you will NEVER get rid of the yeast-related problems.

The end result is that until the yeast condition is addressed, your PMS won't budge. So get on your yeast program and once that improves, get back on the PMS treatment program described earlier in this book.

Low Thyroid

If you want to select a "favorite" hormone for both men and women, the hands down choice is thyroid. Why? Because thyroid has a significant role in just about every metabolic or chemical reaction in the body.

Thyroid deals with a huge range of body physiology. It is involved in everything from fat burning to hair growth. Thyroid influences skin moisture and helps develop a child's brain IQ. So thyroid is vitally important, and without it, you will literally shrivel up and die.

The following are all some of the major symptoms and signs associated with an under active thyroid:

- Depression
- Weight gain
- Difficulty losing weight
- Low energy - fatigue
- Cold natured

- Ice-cold hands or feet
- Dry skin
- Hair loss (alopecia)
- Slowed thinking, poor concentration
- Brain fog
- Memory problems
- Insomnia, poor sleep
- Waking up exhausted
- Tingling in hands and feet
- Muscle pain
- Edema (swelling in ankles)
- Constipation
- Slow heart rate
- Low blood pressure
- Elevated cholesterol
- Thickened tongue
- Anemia
- Thinned eyebrows
- Slow reflexes
- Cool body temperature

However, frank hypothyroidism is not that common. Most of the time when doctors check blood thyroid levels, they usually come back quite "normal". At this point, the doctor will usually tell you that there is "nothing wrong with you" and writes you a prescription for an anti-depressant medication.

Unfortunately, there are significant testing problems with the typical encounter in the doctor's office when it comes to thyroid:

First, the lab values of "normals" are too wide. In other words, the lab has too many people within the normal range. In my observation, about a third of the population should be in the "abnormal" range, particularly over the age of 30. The laboratories used too large a data base to calculate the normal values for a population.

Another problem is the presence of what is called "auto-antibodies" to your own thyroid hormone. The medical name for this is "Hashimoto's Disease". About a third of all women have thyroid anti-bodies and about a sixth of men have them, too.

This means that your body's immune system has somehow been programmed to attack and destroy circulating thyroid hormone in your own body. So the lab can measure all the thyroid hormone it wants, but the end effect of thyroid is not making it inside the cells of the body to start working.

Finally, and this is crucial – your body's ability to manufacture any hormone peaks around the age of 25. After that, hormone manufacturing capability declines at a rate of about 1% - 3% on an annual basis thereafter.

Mathematically, by the time you reach 40, your hormone production could be down as much as 45%.

By your 70th birthday, your hormone production could be just a fraction of what it used to be when you were younger.

This math not only applies to thyroid hormone, but all hormones, including estrogen, progesterone and testosterone, regardless of sex.

The end result is just because your thyroid blood tests were "normal" – don't believe it. There is a very long list of symptoms when your thyroid is under active or deficient.

Therefore, I always add some thyroid hormone to everyone who has intractable PMS, regardless of whether their thyroid blood tests are normal or not.

Where to Get Thyroid?

There are two ways to get thyroid: getting your doctor to write you a prescription for thyroid hormone or get it as a dietary supplement in the form of a thyroid extract.

The best way to get thyroid is to convince your doctor to write a prescription for you. The problem with this is that most doctors will refuse to do this when you test "normal" on your thyroid blood tests.

There is likely not a single mainstream doctor on this planet who will write a thyroid prescription in the face of "normal" blood tests. Progressive doctors who are familiar with bio-identical hormones write thyroid prescriptions nearly 100% of the time, but generally these doctors are very expensive and do not take insurance.

Just for completeness, if your doctor was agreeable to write the thyroid prescription the next problem is that they will universally give you the wrong kind. Doctors love to prescribe a type of thyroid called "T4" or levothyroxine. The brand names for this include: Synthroid, Levothroid, Levoxyl, and Unithroid.

Although you can get away with these brands about half of the time, I do not recommend any of them. Instead, you need a type of thyroid called "T3" or triiodothyronine. The reason why T3 is preferred over T4 is because T3 is the active form of thyroid in the body's cells.

Many people have difficulty converting their T4 into the T3 form. Therefore, any prescription that is exclusively T4 may not be helpful.

We prefer the prescription Armour thyroid. Armour thyroid is an extract that has a combination of T3 with T4. It is far more effective than the T4-only brands.

It must be Brand Name Only for Armour thyroid. No generics!

The prescription that the doctor should write is:
Armour thyroid –
½ grain by mouth on a daily basis for two weeks.

After 2 weeks, increase the dose to 1 grain daily thereafter.

If your doctor is unwilling to prescribe you thyroid medication, then you will have to get it yourself. Here's how:

You can get a dietary supplement version of thyroid extract. Order it off the internet. This is very difficult to find, but my favorite thyroid extract that you can get without a prescription can be found at: http://Thyroid.DepressionGoneForever.com

It is very inexpensive and easy to use.

Recommended Dosage for Thyroid:

The recommended dosage is to take one pill twice daily. The amount of thyroid extract works out at this dose to the equivalent of a half grain of Armour thyroid.

After two weeks, you can double this dose to two capsules, twice daily to become equivalent to the one grain dose of Armour thyroid.

Chronic Fatigue Syndrome/Fibromyalgia

This is another condition that I see that is very common in women who have resistant PMS. I have included both of these conditions together as I believe they are both variations of the same thing.

Chronic Fatigue Syndrome (CFS) is characterized by extreme, profound weakness and fatigue at all times of the day. Some people are so affected that they are almost bedridden. Most people fall into some milder version whereby they run out of gas in the early afternoon. Many people with CFS also have an associated chronic pain condition identical to Fibromyalgia.

Fibromyalgia Syndrome (FMS) is characterized by a chronic pain condition that has numerous tender or trigger points. Mainstream medicine has very specific criteria for diagnosis that requires so many trigger points to qualify. My easy to remember version of FMS is that you have very tender and painful muscles. If someone touches you and you go "ouch", then you have FMS.

People with FMS almost always have a fatigue component strikingly similar to CFS. This is why I maintain that CFS and FMS are basically the variations of the same theme.

New Book on CFS/FMS in 2008

I will be writing another book on this very topic probably early in 2008. There will be more details on theories, explanations and most importantly, how to overcome those conditions. Admittedly, we don't have the "perfect cure" for this condition just yet, but we get pretty close to normalizing people's lives with our unique treatment recommendations.

Unfortunately, the treatment recommendations for CFS/FMS are very complicated and tedious. I will say the basis in treatment lies in the replenishment of adrenal hormones as well as thyroid. This requires a very detailed step-by-step algorithm that we have developed that goes way beyond the scope of this book.

At this point, my recommendation would be to concentrate on the yeast and thyroid issues before plunging into the CFS/FMS arena. That will be several months of experimentation. By that time, my Chronic Fatigue Syndrome/Fibromyalgia book should be ready and you can check that out early next year.

Other Supplements

Before I close, let me comment that regardless of your PMS status, that you (and your family – everyone should be taking these) should be taking the following supplements:

- Multivitamins (with large amounts of B vitamins)

- Krill Oil - this is the latest and best version of omega-3 oil
  (source: http://KrillOil.PMScure.com)

- Vitamin C – at least 3000mg per day

- Calcium – at least 1000 – 1500mg per day

- Magnesium chelates – see prior recommendations: 300 mg/day (source: http://MagnesiumOrder.com)

- Folic Acid – 400 mcg/day

- Vitamin E – 400 IU's/day

- Vitamin D - 400 IU's/day

- Probiotics – Primal Defense

- Kefir – 8 – 16 ounces/day

We recommend other supplements in other specialty situations, but that is beyond the scope of this book.

Conclusion

I hope this helps for the 20% of women who have tried the bio-identical progesterone treatment and failed to get better. It is extremely likely that you saw many of your other health conditions in this chapter and can now act accordingly.

Conclusion

Well, there you have it. PMS is more common than anticipated and have overlapping qualities with other hormonal conditions like migraine headaches, in particular. PMS is probably intimately related to the menstrual cycle and sex hormones in women.

The good news for PMS sufferers out there is that based on our historical treatment rates we can cure about 80% of you. Follow my advice above and **you WILL be cured** with no more PMS for the rest of your life.

For menstruating women, expect about two menstrual cycles to go by to get the full effect and you should not have PMS any more. So, after about 60 days you should be cured.

For non-menstruating women and for men, your cure results can come somewhat quicker.

As I said before, we have an 80% cure rate. For the remaining 20%, many of them may have PMS symptoms caused by something different than sex hormone deficiency, and there is also a small percentage of people with PMS who just don't respond as well to our usual hormone treatment.

Even if you are in the 20% of people whose PMS does not improve, I guarantee that if you follow my program that you will feel better anyway in other areas. Also, your PMS will not be as severe as they were before, even if the source is different from what we thought.

The reason is that correcting hormonal imbalances (or deficiencies) will have an overall positive effect on your health and well-being. You will feel better. Your body will function better. You will stay younger longer. It's all good.

So, good luck. Go order your hormones. Order your Neptune Krill Oil. Don't forget your magnesium and start feeling better in 60 days.

Andrew P. Jones, M.D.

P.S.

Other books by Dr. Jones:

The Natural Cure to Your Migraine Headaches, 2007 Edition – order from www.Migraine-Headaches-Information.com

The All-Natural Cure to Your PMS – order from www.PMScure.com

The All-Natural Cure to Your Depression
– order from www.DepressionGoneForever.com

In my practice of treating women, not only have I come across maladies like depression, but also numerous other problems endemic within the female population.

I have published two other books recently – one on migraine headaches and the other on depression. Both are written in a similar style to this book explaining in common language what these conditions are and how to cure them forever.

To order these books, simply go to my websites listed above or email my office at: help@WomensHealthInstituteofTexas.com or call 281-962-4264.

Disclaimer:

This book represents the views of Dr. Jones alone. It is not intended to allow non-physicians to practice medicine but rather to improve a patient's understanding of their medical condition. Dr. Jones believes that an informed patient can assist better in their own medical care which results in a better outcome for the patient.

This book is not intended for diagnosis but rather to offer information to make you a better informed patient. Discuss any medication changes with your physician prior to making any changes. Please consult your physician for your own personal medical advice.